Defeat Colo-Rectal Cancer

Take control and beat Colo-Rectal Cancer

Dr. Sarah White

Copyright

TABLE OF CONTENT

Introduction

Welcome to "Defeat Colorectal Cancer" by Dr. Sarah White, a comprehensive guide that illuminates the path towards triumph over this formidable adversary. In these pages, Dr. White, a seasoned expert in the field, extends a compassionate hand to those navigating the intricate terrain of colorectal cancer. With a blend of medical expertise and empathetic understanding, this book is a beacon of knowledge and encouragement.

Unveiling the complexities of colorectal cancer, Dr. White delves into the significance of early detection, treatment options, and the ever-powerful role of lifestyle choices. Through a lens of hope and empowerment, readers will discover practical insights and holistic strategies to confront the challenges posed by colorectal cancer head-on. As we embark on this journey together, "Defeat Colorectal Cancer" is not just a guide; it is a roadmap towards resilience, strength, and ultimately, triumph in the face of adversity.

Chapter 1

Understanding Your Diagnosis

In this first chapter, we're going to talk about what it means when you hear that you have colorectal cancer. It might sound a bit complicated, but don't worry—I'm here to help make it clearer for you. We'll break down the important stuff, like what the doctors are looking for and the tests they might do. Understanding your diagnosis is like having a map for your journey through this challenge. By the end of this chapter, you'll know more about what's happening in your body and how you can work with your healthcare team to make the best choices for your health. Let's take this step together and get a better grasp of what's going on.

What is colorectal cancer and how does it affect you

Colorectal cancer is a type of cancer that starts in the colon or rectum, which are parts of the digestive system. The colon and rectum together make up the large intestine.

Causes

Colorectal cancer often begins as small growths called polyps on the inner lining of the colon or rectum. While not all polyps turn into cancer, some can over time. The exact cause of why these changes happen is not always clear, but certain factors can increase the risk:

1. Age: Colorectal cancer is more common in older adults.
2. Family History: If close relatives have had colorectal cancer, it might increase your risk.
3. Lifestyle Factors: Unhealthy habits like a poor diet, lack of physical activity, smoking, and excessive alcohol use can contribute.

Symptoms

Early stages may not show noticeable symptoms, but as the cancer progresses, common signs include changes in bowel habits, blood in stool, abdominal discomfort, fatigue, and unintended weight loss.

Impact

Colorectal cancer affects not only physical health but also emotional well-being. The journey involves medical treatments, lifestyle adjustments, and emotional support. By understanding the causes, recognizing symptoms, and prioritizing regular screenings, individuals can take steps towards early detection and better management of colorectal cancer.

Recognizing Early Signs

Recognizing early signs of colorectal cancer is like paying attention to signals from your body. Here's how to keep an eye out for changes:

1. Watch Your Bathroom Habits:
   - Pay attention to any sudden or persistent changes in how often you go to the bathroom or the way your stool looks.
   - If there's blood in your stool or you notice dark-colored stools, it's essential to let your doctor know.

2. Listen to Your Body:
   - Notice any discomfort or pain in your abdomen, especially if it's new or doesn't go away.

- Unexplained weight loss or fatigue could be signs that something isn't right and should be discussed with your healthcare provider.

3. Be Aware of Your Body's Signals:
   - Trust your instincts. If something feels off or different, it's okay to seek advice.
   - Regular self-checks and awareness of any unusual changes can help catch potential issues early.

4. Know Your Family History:
   - If close family members have had colorectal cancer, inform your doctor. Family history can influence your risk.

5. Don't Ignore Symptoms:
   - Even if you're unsure, it's better to share your concerns with your healthcare team. They can help determine if further investigation is needed.

Remember, understanding what's normal for you and noticing any changes is the first step in recognizing early signs. If something seems unusual, don't hesitate to talk to your healthcare provider. Regular check-ins and open communication are crucial for your well-being.

Common symptoms of colorectal cancer

Recognizing the common symptoms of colorectal cancer involves paying attention to changes in your body. Here are signs that might indicate a need for further evaluation:

1. Changes in Bowel Habits:
   - Persistent diarrhea or constipation without a clear cause.
   - Feeling that your bowel doesn't empty completely.

2. Blood in Stool:
   - Seeing bright red or very dark blood in your stool can be a sign.

3. Abdominal Discomfort:
   - Frequent abdominal cramps, pain, or a feeling of fullness, bloating, or discomfort.

4. Unintended Weight Loss:
   - Losing weight without trying or without changes in diet or exercise.

5. Fatigue:
   - Unexplained tiredness, weakness, or lack of
energy that persists.

6. Iron Deficiency Anemia:
   - Feeling more tired than usual, often due to a low
red blood cell count.

7. Changes in Stool Appearance:
   - Stools that are narrower than usual or have a
different shape.

8. Urgency or Feeling of Incomplete Emptying:
   - Feeling like you need to have a bowel movement
urgently or that you haven't completely emptied
your bowel.

9. Bowel Obstruction Symptoms:
   - Severe cramps, abdominal swelling, and
vomiting, which may indicate a bowel obstruction.

Importance of early detection

Early detection of colorectal cancer is crucial for several important reasons:

1. Improved Treatment Options:
   - Detecting colorectal cancer in its early stages often allows for more effective and less aggressive treatment options. This can include surgery, targeted therapies, and chemotherapy.

2. Increased Chance of Cure:
   - Cancers caught at an early stage have a higher likelihood of being completely cured. Early detection can prevent the cancer from spreading to other parts of the body.

3. Better Quality of Life:
   - Early intervention can lead to less invasive treatments, reducing the impact on a person's daily life and overall well-being.

4. Higher Survival Rates:
   - The survival rate for colorectal cancer is significantly higher when the disease is diagnosed

in its early stages. Regular screenings and prompt action can contribute to improved outcomes.

5. Prevention of Complications:
   - Early detection allows for the removal of precancerous polyps before they turn cancerous, preventing the development of colorectal cancer altogether.

6. Cost-Effective Healthcare:
   - Treating cancer at an early stage can be more cost-effective for both individuals and the healthcare system, as advanced stages often require more extensive and expensive treatments.

7. Quality of Life During Treatment:
   - Detecting cancer early may mean less aggressive treatments, reducing the potential side effects and improving the overall quality of life during and after treatment.

8. Peace of Mind:
   - Regular screenings and early detection provide individuals with peace of mind, knowing that they are taking proactive steps towards their health and well-being.

Overall, the importance of early detection lies in its ability to save lives, improve treatment outcomes, and enhance the overall quality of life for individuals diagnosed with colorectal cancer. Regular screenings and awareness play a key role in achieving these benefits.

III. Screening and Diagnostic Tools

Overview of screening tests (colonoscopy, fecal tests)

Screening tests are like health check-ups for your colon, helping catch potential issues early. Here's a simple overview of two common screening tests:

1. Colonoscopy:
   - Think of it as a thorough inspection of your colon. A doctor uses a flexible tube with a tiny camera to check for polyps (small growths that could turn into cancer) or other abnormalities.
   - It's usually done every 10 years, starting at age 45-50, or earlier if there's a higher risk.

2. Fecal Tests:
   - These are simpler tests that check your stool for signs of colorectal issues.

- a. Fecal Occult Blood Test (FOBT): Detects tiny amounts of blood in the stool that may not be visible. It's usually done annually.
- b. Fecal Immunochemical Test (FIT): Similar to FOBT but specifically detects human blood. Also done annually.

Why Are They Important?

- These tests are vital for early detection. If an issue is found, it can often be treated more effectively, sometimes even preventing cancer from developing.
- Regular screenings, especially for those with higher risk factors, are crucial for maintaining colorectal health.

How to Prepare:

- For a colonoscopy, you may need to adjust your diet and take special medications the day before.
- Fecal tests usually involve collecting a small sample at home and sending it to a lab.

Remember, these screenings are not only for those with symptoms. Regular checks, based on your doctor's recommendations, can help ensure a healthier future.

Understanding the role of diagnostic imaging

Understanding the role of diagnostic imaging in colorectal health is like using special tools to see what's happening inside your body. Here's a simple breakdown:

1. Seeing Inside:
   - Diagnostic imaging involves special machines that take pictures of the inside of your body, helping doctors see details they can't observe from the outside.

2. Colonoscopy:
   - This is like a special camera on a flexible tube that goes through your colon. It helps doctors check for polyps or abnormal growths.

3. CT Scan:
   - Think of it as a high-tech X-ray that creates detailed cross-sectional images. It's useful for detecting tumors and checking if cancer has spread.

4. MRI:

- Like a super-detailed photo machine using magnets and radio waves. It provides clear images of soft tissues, helping doctors understand the extent of the disease.

5. Ultrasound:
   - Uses sound waves to create images. It's helpful for examining the rectum and nearby areas.

6. X-rays:
   - Old but gold. X-rays are like invisible beams passing through your body, helping identify issues like blockages or abnormal growths.

7. Nuclear Medicine:
   - Involves a small amount of radioactive material. It helps track how well organs are functioning.

8. PET Scan:
   - Shows where cells are using more energy. It's helpful in finding areas with increased activity, like cancer cells.

Building a Colorectal-Friendly Diet

Foods to Include

Including nutrient-rich foods during the treatment of colorectal cancer can be beneficial for overall well-being. Here are some foods to consider incorporating into your diet:

1. Lean Proteins:
   - Why: Essential for maintaining muscle mass. Opt for lean protein sources like chicken, fish, tofu, and legumes.

2. Colorful Fruits and Vegetables:
   - Why: Packed with vitamins, minerals, and antioxidants, which support immune function and overall health.

3. Whole Grains:

- Why: Provide energy and essential nutrients. Choose whole grains like brown rice, quinoa, and whole wheat.

4. Fatty Fish:
   - Why: Rich in omega-3 fatty acids, which have anti-inflammatory properties and support heart health.

5. Nuts and Seeds:
   - Why: Provide healthy fats, protein, and various nutrients. Include almonds, walnuts, chia seeds, and flaxseeds.

6. Dairy or Fortified Plant-Based Milk:
   - Why: Excellent sources of calcium and vitamin D, crucial for bone health during treatment.

7. Probiotic-Rich Foods:
   - Why: Support gut health and digestion. Include yogurt, kefir, and fermented foods like sauerkraut.

8. Low-FODMAP Foods:
   - *Why:* For those experiencing digestive symptoms, following a low-FODMAP diet under the guidance of a healthcare professional may be beneficial.

9. Hydration:
   - Why: Staying hydrated is crucial during treatment. Drink plenty of water and consider hydrating foods like water-rich fruits and vegetables.

10. Individualized Nutrition:
   - Why: Work with a registered dietitian to tailor your diet based on your specific needs, taking into account any side effects of treatment.

Foods to avoid

During colorectal cancer treatment, it's often advisable to limit or avoid certain foods that may exacerbate symptoms or interfere with the treatment process. Here are some considerations:

1. Processed Meats
   - Why: Processed meats are linked to an increased risk of colorectal cancer. Opt for lean protein sources like poultry, fish, and plant-based options.

2. Highly Processed Foods:

-Why: Foods high in additives, preservatives, and unhealthy fats may not support overall health during treatment.

3. Excessive Sugary Foods:
   - Why: High sugar intake can contribute to inflammation and may negatively impact immune function.

4. Fried and Greasy Foods:
   - Why: High in unhealthy fats, these can be harder on your digestive system.

5. Spicy Foods:
   - Why: For some individuals, especially those with digestive issues, spicy foods may irritate the stomach or intestines.

6. High-Sodium Foods:
   - Why: Excess sodium can contribute to water retention and may not be suitable for those with certain health conditions.

7. Alcohol:
   - Why: Alcohol can interfere with treatment and may have negative interactions with medications.

8. High-Fiber Foods in Some Cases:
   - Why: For individuals experiencing digestive symptoms, high-fiber foods like raw vegetables or whole grains might be challenging. Consider cooking or choosing lower-fiber options.

9. Dairy Products in Some Cases:
   - Why: Full-fat or high-lactose dairy products may be harder to digest for some individuals. Consider low-fat or lactose-free alternatives.

10. Individualized Nutrition:
   -Why: Work with a registered dietitian to tailor your diet based on your specific symptoms and treatment plan.

Practical Tips for Healthy Eating During Treatment

Maintaining a healthy diet during colorectal cancer treatment is essential for supporting overall well-being. Here are some practical tips to make healthy eating more manageable:

1. Frequent, Smaller Meals:

Why: Eating smaller, more frequent meals can help manage digestive symptoms and maintain energy levels.

2. Stay Hydrated:
   - Why: Hydration is crucial. Sip water throughout the day and consider hydrating foods like water-rich fruits and vegetables.

3. Choose Nutrient-Rich Foods:
   - Why: Opt for whole, nutrient-dense foods to ensure you're getting essential vitamins and minerals.

4. Lean Proteins:
   - Why: Choose lean protein sources like poultry, fish, tofu, and legumes to support muscle health.

5. Manage Fiber Intake:
   - Why: Adjust fiber intake based on your tolerance. Cook vegetables to make them easier to digest, and consider lower-fiber grains.

6. Include Probiotics:
   - Why: Probiotic-rich foods like yogurt can support gut health and digestion.

7. Limit Processed Foods:
   - Why: Minimize intake of highly processed foods, which may contain additives and preservatives.

8. Mindful Eating:
   - Why: Pay attention to hunger and fullness cues. Eating slowly and mindfully can enhance digestion.

9. Experiment with Cooking Methods:
   - Why:bTry different cooking methods, such as steaming or baking, to make foods more palatable and easier to digest.

10. Individualized Approach:
   - Why: Work closely with a registered dietitian to tailor your diet to your specific needs, symptoms, and treatment plan.

11. Address Side Effects:
   - Why: If you experience side effects like nausea or changes in taste, discuss these with your healthcare team to find strategies to manage them.

12. Consider Supplements:
   - Why: If needed, work with your healthcare team to determine if supplements are necessary to fill any nutritional gaps.

Colo-Rectal cancer friendly recipes
1. Ginger Turmeric Carrot Soup

Ingredients
- 1 pound carrots, peeled and chopped
- 1 onion, diced
- 2 cloves garlic, minced
- 1 tablespoon fresh ginger, grated
- 1 teaspoon ground turmeric
- 4 cups low-sodium vegetable broth
- Salt and pepper to taste
- 1 tablespoon olive oil

Instructions
1. In a large pot, heat olive oil over medium heat. Add onions, garlic, and ginger. Sauté until onions are translucent.
2. Add chopped carrots and turmeric. Stir well to coat the carrots with the spices.
3. Pour in the vegetable broth. Bring the mixture to a boil, then reduce heat and simmer until carrots are tender.
4. Use an immersion blender to blend the soup until smooth. Season with salt and pepper to taste.
5. Serve warm, optionally garnished with fresh herbs.

2. Baked Lemon Herb Salmon

Ingredients

- 4 salmon fillets
- 2 tablespoons olive oil
- 2 tablespoons fresh lemon juice
- 1 teaspoon dried dill
- 1 teaspoon dried thyme
- Salt and pepper to taste
- Lemon slices for garnish

Instructions

1. Preheat the oven to 375°F (190°C). Line a baking sheet with parchment paper.
2. Place salmon fillets on the prepared baking sheet.
3. In a small bowl, whisk together olive oil, lemon juice, dill, thyme, salt, and pepper.
4. Drizzle the lemon herb mixture over the salmon fillets, ensuring they are well-coated.
5. Bake in the preheated oven for about 15-20 minutes or until the salmon is cooked through and flakes easily with a fork.

6. Garnish with lemon slices and fresh herbs before serving.

3. Mashed Sweet Potatoes with Cinnamon

Ingredients
- 4 medium-sized sweet potatoes, peeled and cubed
- 2 tablespoons unsalted butter or olive oil
- 1 teaspoon ground cinnamon
- Salt to taste
- Chopped fresh parsley for garnish

Instructions
1. Boil or steam sweet potatoes until tender.
2. Mash the sweet potatoes with butter or olive oil until smooth.
3. Stir in ground cinnamon and add salt to taste.
4. Garnish with chopped fresh parsley before serving.

4. Quinoa and Vegetable Stir-Fry

Ingredients
- 1 cup quinoa, rinsed and cooked according to package instructions

- 2 tablespoons olive oil
- 1 cup broccoli florets
- 1 bell pepper, thinly sliced
- 1 carrot, julienned
- 2 cloves garlic, minced
- Low-sodium soy sauce to taste
- Sesame seeds for garnish

Instructions
1. In a large pan, heat olive oil over medium heat.
2. Add garlic, broccoli, bell pepper, and carrot. Stir-fry until vegetables are tender-crisp.
3. Add cooked quinoa to the pan and mix well.
4. Drizzle with low-sodium soy sauce to taste.
5. Garnish with sesame seeds before serving.

5. Baked Chicken and Sweet Potato Slices

Ingredients
- 4 boneless, skinless chicken breasts
- 2 sweet potatoes, thinly sliced
- 2 tablespoons olive oil
- 1 teaspoon paprika
- 1 teaspoon dried rosemary
- Salt and pepper to taste

Instructions

1. Preheat the oven to 400°F (200°C).
2. Place chicken breasts on a baking sheet.
3. Arrange sweet potato slices around the chicken.
4. Drizzle olive oil over chicken and sweet potatoes.
5. Sprinkle with paprika, dried rosemary, salt, and pepper.
6. Bake for about 25-30 minutes or until the chicken is cooked through and sweet potatoes are tender.

Certainly! Here are two more colorectal cancer-friendly recipes:

6. Butternut Squash and Lentil Soup

Ingredients
- 1 medium butternut squash, peeled and diced
- 1 cup dried green or brown lentils, rinsed
- 1 onion, chopped
- 2 carrots, chopped
- 2 cloves garlic, minced
- 1 teaspoon ground cumin
- 1 teaspoon ground coriander
- 6 cups low-sodium vegetable broth
- Salt and pepper to taste
- Fresh cilantro for garnish

Instructions

1. In a large pot, sauté onions and garlic until softened.
2. Add butternut squash, lentils, carrots, cumin, and coriander. Stir to combine.
3. Pour in vegetable broth and bring to a boil. Reduce heat and simmer until lentils are cooked and vegetables are tender.
4. Use an immersion blender to blend the soup until smooth.
5. Season with salt and pepper to taste.
6. Garnish with fresh cilantro before serving.

7. Grilled Lemon Herb Shrimp Skewers

Ingredients
- 1 pound large shrimp, peeled and deveined
- 2 tablespoons olive oil
- Zest and juice of 1 lemon
- 1 teaspoon dried oregano
- 1 teaspoon dried thyme
- Salt and pepper to taste
- Wooden skewers, soaked in water

Instructions

1. In a bowl, combine olive oil, lemon zest, lemon juice, oregano, thyme, salt, and pepper to create a marinade.
2. Thread shrimp onto soaked skewers.
3. Brush shrimp with the marinade, ensuring they are well-coated.
4. Preheat a grill or grill pan over medium-high heat.
5. Grill shrimp skewers for 2-3 minutes per side or until shrimp are opaque and cooked through.
6. Serve with a side of roasted or steamed vegetables.

Colorectal-friendly snacking options

1. Banana with Almond Butter:
   - Why: Bananas are easy to digest, and almond butter provides healthy fats and protein.

2. Cottage Cheese with Pineapple Chunks:
   - Why: Cottage cheese is a good source of protein, and pineapple adds a sweet and refreshing flavor.

3. Boiled Eggs:
   - Why: Eggs are a protein-rich option that is easy to prepare and digest.

4. Smoothies:
   - Why:bBlend low-fiber fruits like banana and berries with yogurt or lactose-free milk for a nourishing and easy-to-digest snack.

5. Baked Sweet Potato Fries:
   - Why: Sweet potatoes are a good source of vitamins and can be sliced and baked for a tasty, soft snack.

6. Applesauce with Cinnamon:
   - Why: Applesauce is gentle on the digestive system, and cinnamon adds flavor without irritation.

7. Steamed Vegetables with Olive Oil:
   - Why: Steamed vegetables like carrots or zucchini with a drizzle of olive oil provide nutrients in an easily digestible form.

8. Rice Cake with Cream Cheese:
   - Why: Rice cakes are low in fiber, and cream cheese adds a creamy texture with some protein.

9. Yogurt Parfait with Granola:

- Why: Choose low-fat or lactose-free yogurt, layer it with granola, and top with a small amount of berries for a balanced snack.

10. Avocado Toast on White Bread:
   - Why: Avocado is a healthy fat source, and white bread is lower in fiber compared to whole grain options.

11. Grapes with Cheese:
   - Why: Grapes are easy to snack on, and pairing them with a small amount of cheese provides a balance of flavors and textures.

12. Pumpkin Soup:
   - Why: Pumpkin is low in fiber and can be made into a smooth and comforting soup.

Chapter 3

Natural Remedies and Complementary Therapies

Welcome to Chapter 3, where we delve into the realm of "Natural Remedies and Complementary Therapies" in your journey through colorectal health. This chapter explores holistic approaches that complement traditional medical treatments, aiming to enhance overall well-being and support you on a path to recovery. From herbal remedies to mindfulness practices, we'll navigate through a spectrum of strategies that harness the power of nature and alternative therapies. Embrace the possibilities of incorporating these complementary approaches into your routine, recognizing their potential to contribute to your resilience and vitality. Let's embark on a journey where the harmony of natural remedies intertwines with your pursuit of colorectal wellness.

Exploring Natural Healing Approaches

Natural healing approaches encompass a range of holistic practices and complementary therapies that aim to enhance overall well-being and support the body's healing processes. Here are some key components:

1. Herbal Remedies:

   - Description: The use of plants and their extracts for medicinal purposes. Examples include turmeric for its anti-inflammatory properties and ginger for digestive support.
   - Purpose: Herbal remedies are often used to address specific symptoms or support general health.

2. Mindfulness and Meditation

   - Description: Techniques that focus on cultivating present-moment awareness and promoting mental clarity. Practices may include meditation, deep breathing, or mindfulness exercises.
   - Purpose: Reducing stress, anxiety, and promoting emotional well-being.

3. Nutritional Supplements

   - Description: Addition of vitamins, minerals, or other dietary supplements to support overall health.

- Purpose: Addressing potential nutritional deficiencies and promoting optimal health during and after treatment.

4. Acupuncture:
   - Description: Traditional Chinese medicine practice involving the insertion of thin needles into specific points on the body.
   - Purpose: Often used to alleviate pain, nausea, and support overall wellness.

5. Massage Therapy:
   - Description: Hands-on manipulation of soft tissues to enhance relaxation and reduce muscle tension.
   - Purpose: Alleviating physical discomfort, promoting circulation, and supporting mental well-being.

6. Yoga:
   - Description: A mind-body practice involving physical postures, breath control, and meditation.
   - Purpose: Enhancing flexibility, strength, and promoting overall relaxation.

7. Aromatherapy:

- Description: Use of essential oils derived from plants to promote physical and psychological well-being.
 - Purpose: Addressing stress, improving mood, and supporting relaxation.

8. Homeopathy:
 - Description: Treatment based on the principle of "like cures like," where highly diluted substances are used to stimulate the body's natural healing processes.
 - Purpose: Addressing specific symptoms or promoting balance in the body.

9. Chiropractic Care:
 - Description: Focuses on the musculoskeletal system, particularly the spine, to address pain and improve overall health.
 - Purpose: Alleviating discomfort, improving posture, and supporting mobility.

Complementary Therapies to Enhance Well-being

Complementary therapies are holistic practices designed to complement traditional medical treatments, enhancing overall well-being and fostering a more comprehensive approach to health. Here are several complementary therapies that aim to promote well-being:

1. Massage Therapy:

- Description: Hands-on manipulation of muscles and soft tissues to reduce tension, improve circulation, and promote relaxation.

- Purpose: Alleviating physical discomfort, enhancing relaxation, and improving overall mood.

2. Mindfulness Meditation:

- Description: Techniques focusing on cultivating present-moment awareness, often through meditation and mindful breathing.

- Purpose: Managing stress, anxiety, and promoting mental clarity and emotional well-being.

3. Acupuncture:

- Description: Traditional Chinese medicine practice involving the insertion of thin needles into specific points on the body.

- Purpose: Used to address various health concerns, including pain management, stress reduction, and improving energy flow.

4. Yoga:
- Description: A mind-body practice incorporating physical postures, breath control, and meditation.
- Purpose: Enhancing flexibility, strength, and promoting mental and emotional balance.

5. Aromatherapy:
- Description: Use of essential oils extracted from plants to stimulate the senses and promote relaxation or invigoration.
- Purpose: Addressing stress, improving mood, and supporting emotional well-being.

6. Nutritional Counseling:
- Description: Guidance from a registered dietitian or nutritionist to optimize dietary choices for overall health.
- Purpose: Addressing nutritional needs, managing side effects of treatment, and supporting the healing process.

7. Chiropractic Care:

- Description: Focuses on the musculoskeletal system, particularly the spine, to improve alignment and overall well-being.
   - Purpose: Alleviating physical discomfort, enhancing mobility, and improving posture.

8. Biofeedback:
   - Description: A technique that uses electronic monitoring to provide information about physiological processes, allowing individuals to gain better control over bodily functions.
   - Purpose: Managing stress, improving relaxation, and addressing symptoms such as pain.

9. Art or Music Therapy:
   - Description: Creative therapies that use art or music as a means of expression and emotional healing.
   - Purpose: Enhancing emotional well-being, providing an outlet for self-expression, and promoting relaxation.

Chapter 4

Lifestyle Transformations

In Chapter 4, we embark on a transformative journey into "Lifestyle Transformations" designed to empower and enhance your well-being during and after colorectal health challenges. This chapter explores practical changes in daily habits, exercise routines, and stress management strategies. From adopting a colorectal-friendly diet to embracing mindfulness practices, discover the potential for positive shifts that can contribute to a healthier and more fulfilling lifestyle. Let's navigate through the process of transformation, recognizing the profound impact lifestyle choices can have on colorectal health and overall vitality.

Exercise as a Vital Component

Exercise plays a vital role in colorectal cancer treatment, offering numerous physical and mental health benefits. Here's why it's considered a crucial component:

1. Physical Well-being:

- Strength and Endurance: Regular exercise enhances overall strength and endurance, helping individuals better cope with the physical demands of treatment.

- Immune Function: Physical activity supports a healthy immune system, which is essential during colorectal cancer treatment.

- Digestive Health: Exercise can aid digestion and alleviate common gastrointestinal symptoms associated with colorectal cancer and its treatment.

2. Cancer-Related Fatigue Management

- Energy Levels: Engaging in moderate exercise has been shown to reduce cancer-related fatigue, promoting increased energy levels and improved daily functioning.

3. Mental Health Benefits:

- Stress Reduction: Exercise is a powerful stress reliever, helping to reduce anxiety and improve overall mental well-being during the challenges of treatment.

- Mood Enhancement: Regular physical activity releases endorphins, contributing to a more positive mood and a sense of well-being.

4. Maintaining Healthy Body Weight:
- Weight Management: Exercise supports weight management, which is crucial during and after treatment to reduce the risk of complications and support overall health.

5. Enhanced Quality of Life:
- Improved Sleep: Regular exercise can contribute to better sleep patterns, promoting overall quality of life.

- Social Engagement: Group exercises or activities provide an opportunity for social interaction, reducing feelings of isolation and fostering a sense of community.

6. Improved Treatment Tolerance:
- Treatment Side Effects: Exercise may help mitigate certain treatment side effects, such as muscle weakness or joint pain.

7. Cancer Survivorship:

- Reduced Recurrence Risk: Studies suggest that regular exercise may reduce the risk of cancer recurrence and improve long-term outcomes.

It's important to note that the type and intensity of exercise should be tailored to individual capabilities and medical advice. Consult with your healthcare team before starting any exercise program, and work with qualified fitness professionals who have experience with cancer patients.

Whether it's walking, gentle yoga, or strength training, incorporating regular physical activity into your routine can contribute significantly to your overall well-being during colorectal cancer treatment and survivorship.

Exercise routines for colorectal cancer patients should be tailored to individual abilities, taking into account the specific stage of treatment, overall health, and any potential physical limitations. Here are some types of exercise routines that are generally considered suitable for colorectal cancer patients:

Exercise routines

1. Walking:
   - Description: Gentle walking is a low-impact activity that can be adapted to various fitness levels.
   - Benefits: Improves cardiovascular health, helps maintain or improve muscle tone, and contributes to overall well-being.

2. Yoga:
   - Description: Yoga involves gentle stretching, breathing exercises, and relaxation techniques.
   - Benefits: Enhances flexibility, promotes relaxation, and supports mental well-being.

3. Tai Chi:
   - Description: A slow, flowing martial art that involves gentle movements and deep breathing.
   - Benefits: Improves balance, flexibility, and reduces stress.

4. Water Aerobics:
   - Description: Exercise in a pool, which provides buoyancy and reduces impact on joints.
   - Benefits: Enhances cardiovascular fitness, muscle strength, and joint flexibility.

5. Strength Training:

   - Description: Uses resistance to build or maintain muscle strength. Light weights or resistance bands can be used.
   - Benefits:bHelps maintain muscle mass, supports bone health, and improves overall strength.

6. Stationary Cycling:

   - Description: Cycling on a stationary bike is a low-impact exercise that can be adapted to individual fitness levels.
   - Benefits: Improves cardiovascular health, leg strength, and endurance.

7. Gentle Stretching:

   - Description: Incorporates slow and controlled stretching exercises to improve flexibility.
   - Benefits: Helps maintain range of motion, reduces stiffness, and promotes relaxation.

8. Pilates:

   - Description: Focuses on core strength, stability, and controlled movements.
   - Benefits: Enhances core strength, flexibility, and overall body awareness.

9. Breathing Exercises:

- Description: Techniques such as diaphragmatic breathing can be beneficial for relaxation and stress reduction.
- Benefits: Supports respiratory function, reduces anxiety, and enhances overall well-being.

Stress Reduction Techniques

Stress reduction is crucial for colorectal cancer patients, promoting overall well-being and aiding in the coping process. Here are some effective stress reduction techniques:

1. Deep Breathing Exercises:

- Technique: Inhale slowly through your nose, expanding your diaphragm, and exhale slowly through your mouth.
- Benefits: Calms the nervous system, reduces anxiety, and promotes relaxation.

2. Mindfulness Meditation:

- Technique: Focus on the present moment, observing thoughts and sensations without judgment.

- Benefits: Enhances self-awareness, reduces stress, and fosters a sense of tranquility.

3. Progressive Muscle Relaxation (PMR):
   - Technique: Tense and then slowly release different muscle groups, moving from head to toe.
   - Benefits: Relieves muscle tension, promotes relaxation, and reduces physical stress.

4. Guided Imagery:
   - Technique: Visualize calming and positive scenes or experiences.
   - Benefits: Redirects focus, reduces anxiety, and creates a sense of peace.

5. Yoga:
   - Technique: Incorporates physical postures, breathing exercises, and meditation.
   -Benefits: Improves flexibility, reduces stress, and enhances overall well-being.

6. Nature Walks:
   - Technique: Spend time outdoors, connecting with nature through walks or simply sitting in a natural setting.
   - Benefits: Refreshes the mind, reduces stress, and provides a sense of tranquility.

7. Journaling:

- Technique: Write down thoughts, feelings, and experiences.
- Benefits: Provides an emotional outlet, promotes self-reflection, and aids in processing emotions.

8. Listening to Music:

- Technique: Choose calming music and take time to listen mindfully.
- Benefits: Elicits positive emotions, reduces stress, and promotes relaxation.

9. Aromatherapy:

- Technique: Use scents like lavender or chamomile through essential oils or candles.
- Benefits: Calms the senses, reduces anxiety, and enhances relaxation.

10. Social Support:

- Technique: Connect with friends, family, or support groups.
- Benefits: Sharing feelings and experiences can provide emotional support and reduce stress.

11. Laughing Therapy:

- Technique: Engage in activities that bring joy and laughter.
- Benefits: Laughter releases endorphins, reducing stress and improving mood.

12. Massage Therapy:
- Technique: Receive gentle massages to relax tense muscles and promote overall well-being.
- Benefits: Reduces physical tension, enhances relaxation, and provides a sense of comfort.

Prioritizing Quality Sleep for Recovery

Prioritizing quality sleep is crucial for recovery during colorectal cancer treatment. Here are key considerations and tips to enhance sleep:

1. Establish a Consistent Sleep Schedule:
- Routine: Go to bed and wake up at the same time each day, even on weekends, to regulate your body's internal clock.

2. Create a Relaxing Bedtime Routine:
- Preparation: Develop calming activities before bedtime, such as reading, gentle stretching, or practicing relaxation techniques.

3. Optimize Sleep Environment:

- Comfort: Ensure your bedroom is conducive to sleep—comfortable mattress, pillows, and a cool, dark, and quiet environment.

4. Limit Stimulants:

- Caffeine: Avoid caffeinated beverages in the afternoon and evening, as they can interfere with sleep.

5. Mindful Eating:

- Timing: Avoid heavy meals close to bedtime. Consider a light snack if hunger is a concern.

6. Physical Activity:

- Regular Exercise: Engage in regular, moderate exercise, but avoid intense workouts close to bedtime.

7. Manage Stress:

- Relaxation Techniques: Incorporate stress-reducing activities like deep breathing, meditation, or gentle yoga before bedtime.

8. Limit Screen Time:

- Electronic Devices: Reduce exposure to screens
at least an hour before bed, as the blue light emitted
can disrupt sleep.

9. Seek Comfortable Sleep Positions:
- Pain Management: Use pillows or cushions to
support areas of discomfort or surgical sites.

10. Mindful Napping:
- Duration: If you nap during the day, keep it short
(20-30 minutes) to avoid interfering with nighttime
sleep.

11. Hydrate Wisely:
- Timing: Limit fluid intake close to bedtime to
minimize disruptions from bathroom visits.

12. Consult with Healthcare Team:
- Medication: Discuss any sleep disturbances
with your healthcare team, as certain medications or
treatments may impact sleep.

Chapter 5

Empowering Your Mind and Spirit

Welcome to Chapter 5, where we explore "Empowering Your Mind and Spirit" on the road to colorectal health. In this chapter, we'll discover how your thoughts and inner strength play a vital role in facing the challenges of colorectal cancer. By embracing positive perspectives, finding inspiration, and cultivating mindfulness, we aim to empower not just the body but also the mind and spirit in your journey toward well-being. Let's dive into simple yet impactful strategies that connect the power of your thoughts and emotions to your colorectal health, fostering resilience and strength within.

Cultivating a Positive Mindset

Cultivating a positive mindset during your colorectal health journey can significantly impact your well-being. Here are simple yet effective tips to foster a positive outlook:

1. Gratitude Practice:
   - Keep a Journal: Each day, write down three things you're thankful for. It could be as small as a kind gesture or as significant as progress in your treatment.

2. Focus on the Present:
   - Mindfulness: Engage in activities with full attention. Whether it's savoring a meal or taking a gentle walk, be present in the moment.

3. Celebrate Small Victories:
   - Acknowledge Achievements: Recognize and celebrate even the smallest accomplishments. Each step forward, no matter how tiny, is a victory.

4. Surround Yourself with Positivity:
   - Support System: Spend time with people who uplift and encourage you. Positive relationships contribute to a brighter mindset.

5. Affirmations:

- Daily Affirmations: Create positive statements about yourself and your journey. Repeat them regularly to reinforce a positive self-image.

6. Humor and Laughter:
- Find Joy: Incorporate humor into your day, whether through funny movies, jokes, or spending time with those who make you laugh.

7. Set Realistic Goals:
- Achievable Steps: Break down larger goals into smaller, manageable tasks. Achieving these smaller steps can boost your confidence and optimism.

8. Self-Compassion:
Be Kind to Yourself: Treat yourself with the same kindness and understanding you would offer to a friend facing similar challenges.

9. Visualize Success:
- Positive Imagery: Picture yourself overcoming challenges and visualize a positive outcome. This can create a sense of hope and motivation.

10. Learn from Challenges:

- Silver Linings: View challenges as opportunities for growth. Identify lessons or strengths that emerge from difficult situations.

11. Stay Connected:
- Community Engagement: Join support groups or connect with others facing similar journeys. Sharing experiences fosters a sense of community and understanding.

12. Practice Self-Care:
- Prioritize Well-Being: Engage in activities that bring you joy and relaxation. Taking care of yourself contributes to a positive mindset.

Emotional Well-being During Treatment

Maintaining emotional well-being during colorectal cancer treatment is crucial for overall health and resilience. Here are simple tips to nurture your emotional health during this challenging time:

1. Open Communication:
- Express Feelings: Share your thoughts and emotions with trusted friends, family, or a counselor.

Open communication can alleviate emotional burdens.

2. Accept Support:

- Lean on Others: Allow loved ones to provide support. Accepting help can strengthen connections and ease emotional stress.

3. Mindful Breathing:

- Deep Breaths: Practice deep breathing exercises to calm the mind and reduce anxiety. Inhale deeply, hold briefly, and exhale slowly.

4. Positive Affirmations:

- Encouraging Words: Repeat positive affirmations to counter negative thoughts. Remind yourself of your strength and resilience.

5. Creative Outlets:

- Express Yourself: Engage in creative activities like writing, art, or music to express emotions and find solace.

6. Establish Routines:

- Predictable Structure: Create daily routines to bring a sense of predictability, which can be comforting during uncertain times.

7. Set Realistic Expectations:

- Manage Goals: Establish achievable expectations for yourself. Break down tasks into manageable steps to reduce stress.

8. Mindful Eating:

- Nourish Your Body: Pay attention to your nutrition. Eating well contributes to both physical and emotional well-being.

9. Connect with Nature:

- Outdoor Time: Spend time in nature for a refreshing break. Whether it's a short walk or simply sitting outside, nature can have a calming effect.

10. Seek Professional Support:

- Therapeutic Guidance: Consider talking to a mental health professional who specializes in cancer-related issues for additional support.

11. Stay Informed:

- Knowledge Empowers: Stay informed about your treatment plan. Understanding what to expect can alleviate uncertainties and fears.

12. Mindful Rest:

- Quality Sleep: Prioritize good sleep hygiene. A well-rested mind is better equipped to handle emotional challenges.

Remember, it's normal to experience a range of emotions during treatment. Be patient with yourself and allow the time and space needed for healing. If emotions become overwhelming, seek support from your healthcare team or a mental health professional. Prioritizing emotional well-being alongside physical health contributes to a more comprehensive and resilient approach to colorectal cancer treatment.

Chapter 6

Navigating Treatment Side Effects Naturally

Welcome to Chapter 6, where we embark on a journey of "Navigating Treatment Side Effects Naturally." In this chapter, we explore gentle and holistic approaches to managing the side effects associated with colorectal cancer treatment. From addressing fatigue to alleviating nausea, we'll delve into natural strategies that complement medical interventions, promoting comfort and well-being. Let's navigate the path of minimizing treatment side effects with mindful choices, acknowledging the body's resilience, and fostering a sense of balance during this challenging but transformative phase of your colorectal health journey.

Managing Common Side Effects

Managing common side effects during colorectal cancer treatment is essential for maintaining overall well-being. Here are simple tips to help address some of the most common side effects:

1. Fatigue:
- Balanced Rest: Prioritize adequate rest without overexertion. Break tasks into smaller, manageable segments, and listen to your body's signals.

2. Nausea and Digestive Issues:
- Ginger: Consider incorporating ginger into your diet, whether through tea, supplements, or ginger candies. It's known for its anti-nausea properties.

3. Appetite Changes:
- Small, Frequent Meals: Opt for smaller, more frequent meals to manage changes in appetite. Include nutrient-dense foods for sustained energy.

4. Mouth Sores:
- Gentle Oral Care: Use a soft toothbrush and mild toothpaste. Rinse your mouth with a saltwater solution to promote healing and reduce discomfort.

5. Hair Loss:
- Comfortable Headwear: If experiencing hair loss, consider comfortable headwear options like scarves

or hats. Choose what makes you feel confident and at ease.

6. Skin Sensitivity:
   - Gentle Skincare: Use fragrance-free, gentle skincare products to soothe sensitive skin. Stay hydrated and protect your skin from excessive sun exposure.

7. Coping with Stress:
   - Mindfulness: Engage in mindfulness practices to manage stress. Deep breathing, meditation, or gentle yoga can contribute to emotional well-being.

8. Peripheral Neuropathy:
   - Comfortable Footwear: Opt for comfortable footwear and consider gentle exercises like foot stretches to alleviate discomfort associated with peripheral neuropathy.

9. Coping with Anxiety:
   - Therapeutic Activities: Explore therapeutic activities such as art, music, or journaling to cope with anxiety. Expressing your feelings creatively can provide emotional relief.

10. Pain Management:

- Communication with Healthcare Team: Communicate openly with your healthcare team about any pain or discomfort. They can adjust medications or suggest alternative approaches to manage pain effectively.

11. Maintaining Hydration:
- Hydrating Beverages: Stay well-hydrated with clear and soothing beverages. Sip water, herbal teas, or broths throughout the day.

Natural Remedies to Alleviate Discomfort

Natural remedies can complement medical interventions in alleviating discomfort associated with colorectal cancer treatment. Here are simple and natural approaches to consider:

1. Ginger for Nausea:
- Usage: Incorporate ginger into your diet through ginger tea, chews, or as a seasoning. Its anti-nausea properties may help alleviate queasiness.

2. Peppermint for Digestive Issues:

- Usage: Sip peppermint tea to ease digestive discomfort. Peppermint oil capsules may also be considered under guidance.

3. Aloe Vera for Skin Sensitivity:

- Usage: Apply pure aloe vera gel to soothe sensitive or irritated skin. Ensure it's free from additives or fragrances.

4. Chamomile for Relaxation:

- Usage: Chamomile tea can promote relaxation and ease stress. Enjoy a cup before bedtime for its calming effects.

5. Turmeric for Inflammation:

- Usage: Incorporate turmeric into your diet. Its active compound, curcumin, has anti-inflammatory properties that may help manage inflammation.

6. Acupressure for Nausea:

- Usage: Explore acupressure wristbands, designed to alleviate nausea by applying pressure to specific points on the wrist.

7. Lavender for Stress Relief:

 - Usage: Lavender essential oil in a diffuser or added to a carrier oil for gentle massage may help reduce stress and promote relaxation.

8. Oatmeal Baths for Skin Comfort:
 - Usage: Soothe irritated skin with colloidal oatmeal baths. Add finely ground oatmeal to warm bathwater for relief.

9. Essential Oils for Anxiety:
 - Usage: Essential oils like lavender, chamomile, or frankincense, when diffused or diluted for topical use, can contribute to a calming atmosphere.

10. Probiotics for Digestive Health:
 - Usage: Incorporate probiotic-rich foods like yogurt or consider probiotic supplements to support gut health and manage digestive issues.

11. Acupuncture for Pain Relief:
 - Usage: Explore acupuncture as a complementary therapy for pain relief. Ensure it's performed by a qualified and experienced practitioner.

12. Warm Compress for Peripheral Neuropathy:

- Usage: Apply a warm compress to areas experiencing peripheral neuropathy. Ensure it's not too hot, and use it for short durations to alleviate discomfort.

Chapter 7

Personal Stories of Resilience

Connecting Through Shared Experiences

In the quiet town of Oakridge, Shared, a resilient soul with a contagious smile, found herself facing an unexpected adversary – colorectal cancer. Her journey through diagnosis, treatment, and triumph over the disease would become a testament to courage, community, and the power of resilience.

It all began one autumn afternoon when Shared started experiencing persistent abdominal discomfort. Initially dismissing it as minor digestive issues, she soon realized that something more profound might be at play. With a mixture of trepidation and determination, she scheduled a visit to her family doctor, Dr. Patterson.

After a series of tests and screenings, the results were delivered with a weight that seemed to suspend time. Shared had been diagnosed with colorectal cancer. The news was a seismic shock, shaking the very foundations of her world. Fear and uncertainty loomed large, but within the depths of Shared's spirit, a quiet strength began to emerge.

Dr. Patterson, with unwavering compassion, explained the treatment options ahead. Shared's journey into the world of chemotherapy, surgeries, and the unknown began. Yet, amidst the clinical protocols and medical intricacies, she discovered an unexpected source of strength – the Oakridge community.

Neighbors, friends, and even acquaintances rallied around Shared, forming a collective shield of support. Meals appeared on her doorstep, friends took turns accompanying her to treatments, and a dedicated group organized fundraisers to alleviate the financial burden that often accompanies a cancer diagnosis. The town, it seemed, had become an extended family, each member contributing a thread to the tapestry of Shared's healing.

As the chemotherapy sessions commenced, Shared's indomitable spirit shone through. She adorned her bald head with vibrant scarves, turning a symbol of vulnerability into one of resilience. The Oakridge community, deeply moved by her grace and strength, reciprocated by organizing a head-shaving event, demonstrating solidarity in the face of adversity.

Throughout the process, Shared's perspective on life underwent a profound transformation. She discovered an inner wellspring of gratitude for the seemingly ordinary moments – a warm cup of tea, the embrace of a loved one, or the rustle of leaves in her backyard. Cancer had not stolen these joys; rather, it had illuminated their significance.

Shared's journey also revealed the importance of mental and emotional well-being. Mindfulness practices, supported by the local cancer support group, became integral to her routine. Guided meditations and shared stories with fellow warriors forged connections that transcended the physical challenges they faced.

The pivotal moment arrived when Shared underwent surgery to remove the cancerous growth. The community, ever-present in their support, organized a "Healing Tree" ceremony. Each resident tied a ribbon to a tree in Shared's yard, symbolizing their collective hope and positive energy for her recovery. It was a visual testament to the interconnectedness of a community determined to see one of their own emerge victorious.

Post-surgery, as Shared embarked on the path of recovery, she realized that cancer had not defined her; rather, it had become a chapter in the larger narrative of her life. The Oakridge community, having walked alongside her through the darkest valleys, now celebrated her triumphant return to health.

The story of Shared's victory over colorectal cancer became a beacon of hope in Oakridge. It inspired an annual community event – the "Shared Walk for Resilience." Residents, young and old, walked together in solidarity, not just for Shared but for every person navigating the challenging terrain of cancer.

Shared's journey left an indelible mark on Oakridge. It was a story not just of survival but of thriving – of a community that transformed fear into fortitude, adversity into unity, and illness into an opportunity for collective healing. Shared, with her radiant smile, had become a living testament to the extraordinary strength that emerges when a community stands together in the face of life's greatest challenges.

Chapter 8

Planning for Life After Treatment

Gradual Transitions to Normalcy

Gradual transitions to normalcy after facing health challenges, such as colorectal cancer, require thoughtful consideration and a holistic approach. Here's a roadmap for easing back into a semblance of normal life:

1. Physical Recover
   - Progressive Activities: Gradually reintroduce physical activities based on your energy levels. Begin with gentle exercises and slowly increase intensity as your strength improves.

2. Nutritional Rehabilitation
   - Balanced Diet: Continue to prioritize a balanced diet rich in nutrients. Work with a nutritionist to address any dietary modifications made during

treatment and gradually reintegrate a variety of foods.

3. Emotional Well-Being:

- Therapeutic Support: Engage in ongoing emotional support, whether through counseling, support groups, or individual therapy. Addressing the emotional aftermath is crucial for a smooth transition.

4. Regular Check-ups:

- Health Monitoring: Maintain regular check-ups with your healthcare team to monitor your recovery progress and address any lingering concerns or potential side effects.

5. Gradual Return to Work:

- Flexible Schedule: If applicable, discuss a gradual return to work with your employer. Consider a part-time schedule or flexible hours to ease back into professional responsibilities.

6. Social Reintegration:

- Reconnect Socially: Reconnect with friends and family at a pace that feels comfortable. Social interactions can be emotionally fulfilling and contribute to a sense of normalcy.

7. Mindfulness Practices:

- Continued Techniques: Continue practicing mindfulness and relaxation techniques. These habits established during treatment can support ongoing emotional well-being.

8. Celebrating Milestones:

- Acknowledge Progress: Celebrate milestones in your recovery journey, whether big or small. It could be completing a physical challenge, reaching a certain emotional milestone, or marking anniversaries.

9. Re-establishing Hobbies:

- Rediscover Interests: Reintroduce hobbies and activities you enjoyed before your health challenges. Engaging in familiar activities can bring a sense of normalcy and joy.

10. Family and Caregiver Communication:

- Open Dialogues: Maintain open communication with your family and caregivers. Share your feelings, expectations, and any concerns as you navigate the transition.

11. Setting Realistic Expectations:

- Patient Self-Compassion: Be patient with yourself and set realistic expectations. Understand that the process of returning to normalcy is gradual and unique to each individual.

12. Physical Fitness Routine:

- Tailored Exercise: Work with a fitness professional to develop a tailored exercise routine that aligns with your current health status and gradually increases in intensity.

13. Counseling Support:

-Post-Treatment Counseling: Consider post-treatment counseling to address any psychological adjustments. This can help process the experience and develop coping strategies for life after cancer.

14. Reconnecting with Passions:

- Passion Pursuits: Reconnect with passions or discover new interests. Engaging in activities that bring joy and fulfillment contributes to a sense of normalcy.

15. Reflecting on the Journey:

- Personal Reflection: Take time to reflect on your journey, acknowledging the challenges faced and the resilience displayed. This reflection can foster a sense of closure and gratitude.

The transition to normalcy is a personalized journey, and there is no one-size-fits-all approach. Listen to your body, communicate openly with your support network, and embrace the gradual reintegration into everyday life with patience and self-compassion.

Long-term Lifestyle Strategies for Colorectal Health

1. Balanced Diet:
   - Fiber-Rich Foods: Incorporate fruits, vegetables, whole grains, and legumes into your diet. High-fiber foods contribute to bowel regularity and overall digestive health.

2. Hydration:
   - Adequate Water Intake: Stay well-hydrated by drinking plenty of water throughout the day. Proper hydration supports healthy digestion and helps prevent constipation.

3. Limit Red and Processed Meats:

- Moderation: Limit the consumption of red and processed meats. Opt for lean protein sources such as fish, poultry, beans, and nuts.

4. Regular Physical Activity:

- Exercise Routine: Engage in regular physical activity. Aim for at least 150 minutes of moderate-intensity exercise per week. Exercise supports overall health and can reduce the risk of colorectal cancer.

5. Maintain a Healthy Weight:

- Balanced Lifestyle: Strive for a healthy weight through a combination of a balanced diet and regular exercise. Obesity is linked to an increased risk of colorectal cancer.

6. Limit Alcohol Consumption:

- Moderation: If you consume alcohol, do so in moderation. Excessive alcohol intake is associated with a higher risk of colorectal cancer.

7. Tobacco Cessation:

- Quit Smoking: If you smoke, consider quitting. Smoking is linked to various cancers, including colorectal cancer.

8. Regular Screenings:

- Routine Check-ups: Adhere to recommended colorectal cancer screenings based on your age and risk factors. Early detection can significantly improve outcomes.

9. Sun Protection:

- UV Protection: Protect your skin from harmful UV rays by using sunscreen, wearing protective clothing, and avoiding excessive sun exposure. Some studies suggest a link between sunburns and an increased risk of colorectal cancer.

10. Stress Management:

- Relaxation Techniques: Practice stress-reducing activities such as deep breathing, meditation, or yoga. Chronic stress may impact digestive health.

11. Limit Processed Foods:

- Whole Foods Focus: Minimize the consumption of processed and refined foods. Focus on a diet rich in whole, nutrient-dense foods.

12. Regular Health Check-ups:

- Comprehensive Exams: Beyond colorectal cancer screenings, schedule regular check-ups with your healthcare provider to monitor overall health.

Adopting these long-term lifestyle strategies can contribute to maintaining colorectal health and reducing the risk of colorectal cancer. It's essential to tailor these recommendations to your individual health status, and consulting with healthcare professionals can provide personalized guidance for your well-being.

Conclusion

Dear Valued Readers,

I am deeply grateful for your support in choosing "Defeat Colorectal Cancer" as a companion on your journey to colorectal health. Writing this book has been a labor of love, fueled by the desire to provide guidance, encouragement, and practical insights for individuals navigating the complexities of colorectal cancer.

As you delve into the pages, I hope you find valuable information that empowers you in your pursuit of well-being. Your health is paramount, and it's my sincere wish that this book serves as a source of knowledge and inspiration.

If you discover the content to be helpful on your path to defeating colorectal cancer, I kindly request your support in leaving a review. Your reviews not only provide feedback but also contribute to the visibility of the book, enabling it to reach and assist more individuals in need.

Thank you for entrusting me with a role in your health journey. Your strength, resilience, and commitment to well-being are truly commendable. May your path be filled with healing, support, and the realization of a brighter, healthier future.

Wishing you good health and a journey filled with triumphs,

Dr. Sarah White

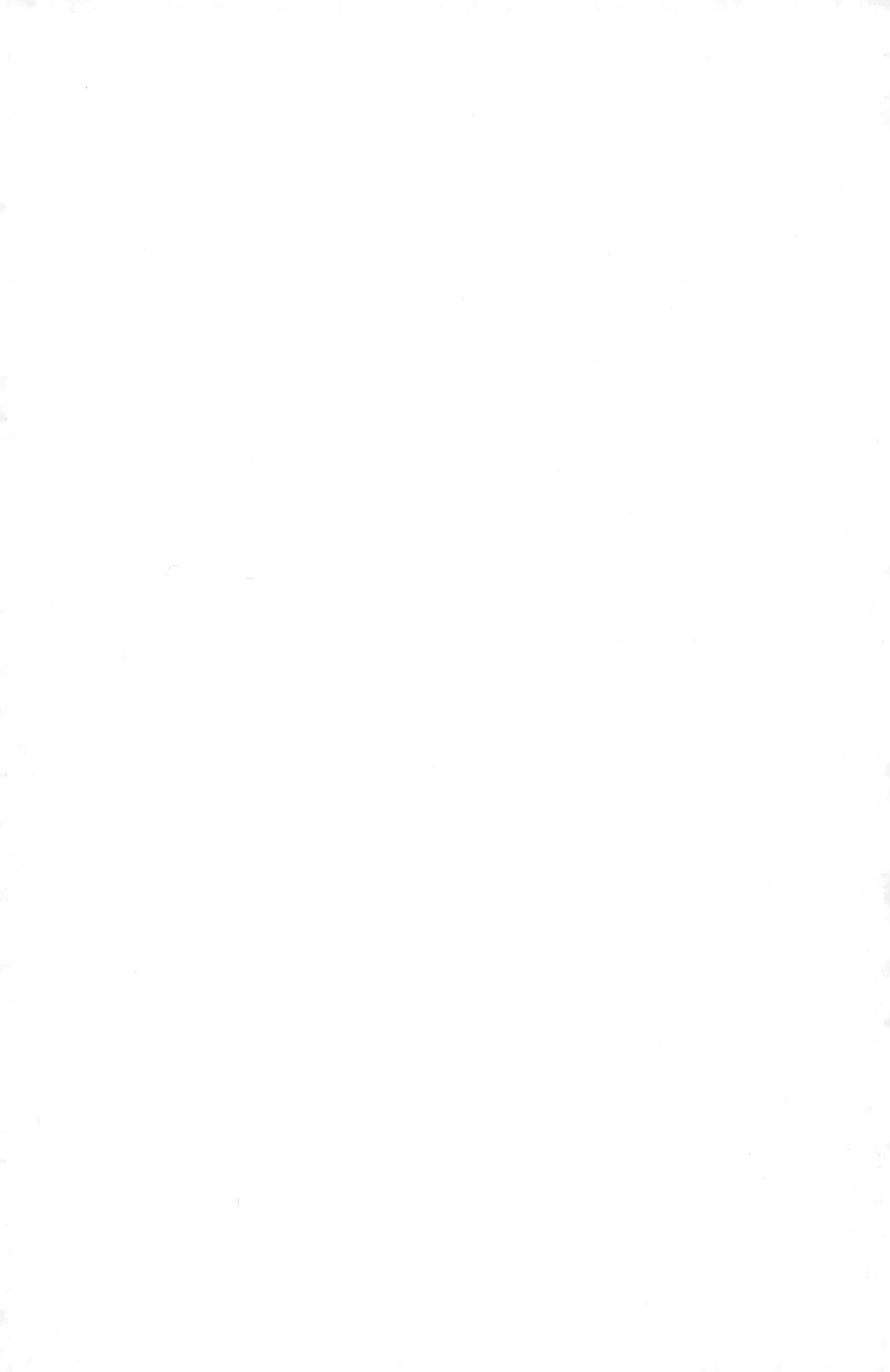